Ultimate Running Weight Loss Guide!

Running

Awesome Highly Effective Running Workouts To Burn Fat Fast, Build Lean Muscle And Increase Your Metabolism To Get In Shape!

Sarah Brooks

Copyright © 2014 Sarah Brooks

Legal Notice

Disclaimer Notice

Table Of Contents

Introduction

I want to thank you and congratulate you for purchasing the book, *Running: Ultimate Running Weight Loss Guide! Awesome Highly Effective Running Workouts To Burn Fat Fast, Build Lean Muscle, And Increase Your Metabolism To Get In Shape!"*

This book contains proven steps and strategies on how to lose weight thru running. More importantly, losing weight is only one of the benefits you will derive from running on a regular basis. By following the guidelines provided in this eBook, your general health will also improve i.e. cardiovascular, skeletal, nervous system, as well as mental acuity. Fat and flab should also give way to muscle. If you do this correctly, then your flabby body will become sleek and toned.

This eBook focuses on effectivity and efficiency. The former refers to doing the right things in order to lose the flab. The latter refers to working smarter, in order to target specific problem areas. For example, a lean but flabby body requires a different type of workout as opposed to an obese individual. Medical preconditions should also be considered.

Think of this eBook as a lifestyle change. You need to assess and then reconfigure the way you live in order to make the most out of each workout. This eBook will focus on 3 key points.

Why should you Believe Me?

I am not an athlete who can train several hours a day with a whole team of nutritionists, and the bottomless food allowance provided by sponsors. I am not a millionaire who can leisurely go to the track to work out. I don't have a nutritionist/cook to prepare my meals for me. I am, however, a competitive runner.

I am an ordinary Joe, aged 45, with a passion for fitness. I have a full time job so I can only workout 1 hour a day at most during the weekdays and 2, sometimes 3 hours during the weekends. I like to eat takeout, fried foods and pizza; but I do this in moderation. I have finished in the podium in several local running, duathlon, and triathlon events. This means I run 6 to 7 minute miles on long distances, a lot faster during shorter distances.

It took me 4 maybe 5 years to get to this point (165 pounds). Before that, I was an overweight individual. I was 5 feet 10 inches and weighed around 280 pounds, mostly fat and flab. For my height, a healthy weight should be around 150 to 180 pounds. Part of the delay was because I did a lot of experimentation. I had a couple of injuries due to inexperience and sheer stupidity. By my reckoning, if I knew then what I know now, I could have probably done this faster and made it more enjoyable.

To be clear, this eBook is not here to show you how to run 6 minute miles. Although, that will come in time, provided you stay true to the teachings in this eBook, for say 2 years. Save that for your long-term goal. This eBook is here to show you how to get off the couch, slim down and change fat with muscle in 3 to 6 months.

This means you no longer wheeze when you walk from the living room to your garage. You no longer have to stop midway in a flight of stairs. You no longer have a protruding belly that obstructs the view to your one eyed snake. Heck, I was obese for more than 5 years! This meant that my large below obstructed by view from the waist down. 5 bloody years! Heck, I could have declared my one eyed monster legally dead after not seeing it for that long!

Thanks again for purchasing this book, I hope you enjoy it!

Chapter 1: Running Basics For Fat Loss

Man was born to walk and to run. Generally speaking, there are 3 steps to running: put 1 foot over the other; then the other foot; now repeat at a fast pace. It's that easy!

For the purposes of this eBook, we will concentrate on low intensity to medium intensity runs. This will comprise around 90% of your running menu. The remaining 10% will be speed form, just to give you a taste of how fast you can go and how fast you've become. Because yes, we know, if someone is beside you, you're racing!

Health Check First

Get a complete physical examination. Tell your doctor you want to run in order to lose weight. In doing so, you can get professional advice and/or a clean bill of health.

Low to Medium Intensity for Weight Loss

Studies have shown that the type of fuel you burn depends on how fast your heart rate is. Incidentally, the faster your heart rate, the faster you are running and vice versa. Simply put, humans use 2 types of fuel. In most cases, we use both at the same time. It is the ratio of fat to carbohydrates used that is important!

The first type is carbohydrate. Take note, carbohydrates provide our body with the energy to move. This is the preferred fuel that our body uses for high intensity running. To put it bluntly, high intensity running means you run balls out with your ugly face on! In terms of heart rate, this means 85% to 98% of your maximum heart rate. In which case, you consume more carbohydrates than you consume fat. The problem is by consuming more carbohydrates, you tend to burn out faster without really utilizing your fat deposits.

The second type of fuel is fat. Our body prefers to use more fat only when we are doing low to medium intensity workouts. Simply put, this means you can hold a conversation while running. Your voice does not stutter. You do not wheeze when breathing. This is equivalent to around 60% to 80% of your maximum heart rate.

Therefore, by running at low to moderate intensity, we are able to target the fat, as opposed to burn you out.

Proper Running Form and Weight Loss

The most important part of running to lose weight is to run injury free. Think about it. If you get injured, you'll probably have to forego running for a week to a month, or even more. That isn't going to help you lose weight!

Proper Breathing

Breathe in with your nose and out with your mouth. Breathe in when your foot hits the ground and out when you are in the air. Breathe as naturally as possible. Not too deep, not too shallow. At slow and moderate speeds, this means your breathing does not slur the way you talk. Take regular breathes. Breathe with your stomach NOT with your shoulders.

Mid-foot Landing

There has been much debate about heel strikers and mid-foot strikers. Without going into the detail, suffice it to say that ALL elite runners land on their mid-foot. So you should too!

Proper Posture

Run straight (not bending forward and/or backward), shoulders, arms and thighs relaxed. Never slouch or puff your chest out while running because this will obstruct your airway. Pay attention to this especially when you get tired.

Arm Movement

Let your arms swing naturally. Shoulders should not be bunched up nor sag low. Keep it at a neutral position. Arms should be bent at the elbow. Don't raise your lower arms to your chest. Arms standby position should be kept low so that your wrists are side by side with your waist. Now move it up and down back and forth in as natural a manner as possible, keeping in tune with your foot stride and speed.

Raise Knees

Never collapse your knee when hitting the ground while running. This will result in knee pain and injury. When your foot hits the ground, it should be right below your waist, never in front of it. You want your foot and knee to land and spring up diagonally. This maximizes shock absorption, gravity use, and minimizes braking motion that puts more pressure on your knees.

Gravity Helps

Stand straight. Now lean slightly forward. You want to find that point where you lean but don't fall. By running with a slight diagonal lean (not slouching), you use gravity to propel you forward.

Run Like a Gazelle

Traditional running form is known as the gazelle. Simply put, you increase the distance you take between each step by following thru with the foot touching the ground and propelling yourself upwards diagonally. The result is your back foot ends up extended backwards and your front foot has the knee raised and lower leg diagonally positioned, with your foot slightly bent low pointing to the ground. As a result you increase distance and minimize the steps you take. This means maximum trust and minimal braking.

Chapter 2: Get In shape With Proper Running Gear

Running requires very little gear. All you really need are appropriate clothes for the weather. Most important of all, you need the perfect pair of shoes for your foot type and running gait.

Avoid buying shoes online unless you already have a pair, or they've got a no questions asked return policy. The best way to buy shoes is to go to a sports outlet that specializes in running, with a running gait analyzer. Don't worry almost every running has it now. This will allow you to determine the best running shoe for you. Try it on and walk several meters. If you feel that something hurts, then find something else. Why? This is because, if it hurts after several meters, then it will hurt much more after several kilometers.

Running Outfit

For warm climates you want a sleeveless shirt and a pair of shorts. For cold climates, you should layer a t-shirt with a sweat shirt and sweat pants. No need to buy expensive brands. All you need is a comfortable pair. Although, you can invest in dry fit or technical clothes as a reward, say after completing the first 2 months of training. Buy items on sale!

Running Gadgets

There are plenty of gears that are being sold nowadays. If you are running at night, then invest in reflective gear and a running light. That is a must! No need to buy expensive hydration bottles. Just bring a simple PET container, preferably with handle.

Distance Meter

GPS watches are expensive. For now, you don't need it. If you have a smart phone, and chances are you do, then download running applications. This allows you to count your steps, distance and speed. How is this possible? Simple, most smart phones nowadays have a GPS chip and accelerometer.

Heart Rate Monitors

Unless you have a heart condition or your doctor advices you do get one from the very start, there is really no need for a heart rate monitor just yet. Granted, it is a useful gadget, especially when paired with your GPS phone; but it is a luxury, not a necessity. Of course, if you do plan to buy a gadget as a reward for yourself, for say, finishing a 5-kilometer fun run below 30 minutes, then a heart rate monitor that pairs via Bluetooth 4.0, with your smartphone should be your first buy. This allows you to really tune up your running to a specific heart rate zone and percentage for maximum fat burning.

Chapter 3: Warm Up And Cool Down

More often than not, inexperienced runners go to the track, road, treadmill, trail, etc., and start to run without even warming up and/or stretching. What is worst is that some individuals choose to run at full throttle at the get go. This is a big mistake. Your muscles aren't ready to cope with the added stress. By analogy, it's like driving your manual speed automobile and shifting from neutral to third gear.

Best case scenario, you're going to experience muscle pain over your legs. Your back and shoulders are going to feel stiff. You might even experience side stitches. After a few minutes, these inexperienced runners get winded and brake to a complete stop. They then find a chair or go to the side of the street and sit down. After 5 minutes, they try to stand up and they get cramps. Worst case scenario, you'll injure yourself.

Warm Up

Warm up comes before you stretch. This allows you to increase blood flow all over your body. This is a signal to your muscles to prepare for the added strain. Since you are running, then the best warm up for you is to walk. Typically, you should walk for 10 minutes. At the 5-minute mark, you should level up to brisk walking; and then slowdown 1 minute before your warm up ends.

Incorporated Dynamic Stretching

After the 10-minute mark on your warm up, perform leg lunges while walking. Alternate between walking and lunges 1 minute at a time, until you hit the 3-minute mark. Now slow down, stretch your shoulders and arms. After 2 minutes, stop and stretch your back. All done!

Cool Down

Cooling down is simply walking 5 to 10 minutes after you finish running. You might be tempted to stop and sit after your run. Avoid this. It is best to walk slowly and deliberately. This way you flush out all the excess lactic acid in your system and allow your body to get used to the lower strain.

Chapter 4: Proper Diet For Faster Weight Loss

The popular misconception is: you run on an empty stomach. Then you eat whatever you want afterwards. In reality, you need to eat before you run and you have to watch what you eat after.

Balanced Diet

You need to eat 3 healthy meals a day. Eat proper portions, appropriate for your weight. The best way to do this is to consult a nutritionist. Make sure to tell him/her that you are running to lose weight.

Pre Run Eats

You need to eat 1 hour before you run. Prioritize easy to digest carbohydrates that you can use as fuel. The top 5 pre run meals are as follows:

- Peanut butter sandwich
- 6 to 8 ounces of oatmeal
- 6 to 8 ounces of sweet potato or yam
- 1 piece banana
- Ugali (boiled corn flour paste)

Avoid eating dairy products, sugar, fried foods, fiber-rich fruits and protein-rich foods. These foodstuff make you feel heavy and can even cause you to feel side stitches.

Pre-race Fluids

Take the recommended 8 glasses of water for the whole day. Add to that, 8 ounce of water 1 hour before. And 4 to 6 ounces of water immediately before you run.

Eating and Drinking while Running

Unless it is an extremely hot and humid day, you do not need to bring water for runs that don't exceed 1 hour. You can if you want to, and you should probably drink 2 to 4 ounces per kilometer. For runs that exceed 1 hour, then you drink to thirst, but not more than 4 to 6 ounces of water per kilometer.

After Run Eats and Drinks

A banana and some chocolate milk will do you some good. Eat the same within 30 minutes after you run. You can also drink 12 to 16 ounces of water. Tip: You can increase and decrease water intake post run using your weight as a basis. Weigh yourself before the run. Now weigh yourself after the run. The trick is to be the same weight before and after the run. That's where post-race eats and drinks come in. Not to worry, you'll still be lighter each morning.

Meal After

The main meal (breakfast, lunch, dinner) after your run is very important. Yes, you can eat a little bit more, but in moderation, and make sure to eat the right types of food. Remember: always have a larger serving of veggies and fruits as opposed to meat. If possible, it is better to eat poultry and fish as opposed to pork and beef. That is why it is a good idea to run before breakfast. This is because, breakfast can be the heartiest meal of the day, and your body has the time to fully digest and utilize what you've eaten. This is as opposed to running late afternoon and eating a heavy meal at night.

Chapter 5: Running Workouts To Increase Your   Metabolism

For best results you need different type of running exercises. This not only targets different muscle groups, it also makes running more fun. Below are a few things you need to understand.

Run 3 to 4 Times a Week

If you want to lose weight, then you need to rack up on mileage. Run on alternate days i.e. Monday, Wednesday, Friday, Sunday, Tuesday, Thursday, Saturday. By doing so, you push just enough but still allow your body to recuperate.

Tip: Everybody is busy; but somewhere somebody who is busier than you is working out! Find the time! Schedule it and actually be there!

Trail vs. Road vs. Treadmill

The best running surface is a relatively flat and well-travelled trail. This minimizes the shock that your body is subjected to. If there are no safe trails, then choose roads. Just make sure to run on the shoulder and against traffic. You want to see the vehicles coming towards you. Treadmill training is also okay, but it's the most boring of them all.

Easy Run

You want 1 easy run per week. An easy run is performed below your moderate pace, and at the shortest distance per week. Simply put, you can talk to the person beside you for long periods of time while running. This pace is just a little bit above brisk walking pace.

Interval Run

An interval run can be easy or hard. Easy intervals require you to run at a fast pace for a minute or two and slow down for long periods of time i.e. 3 to 6 minutes. A hard interval run is the reverse. You run hard for a longer time and you rest for a shorter time. You should perform 1 easy interval run per week.

LSD Run

Once a week, preferably during one of your off days, you perform a long distance run. Don't worry, the pace will be slow. The goal is to run at low intensity at maximum distance in order to increase fat burn!

10% Rule

As a rule of thumb, never increase intensity and /or mileage by more than 10% per week. In other words, you can run longer and faster the following week, but not to the extent that it is more than 10% from the week before. This is important to ensure that your body can keep up with the demands you put it thru!

Sample Training Program

Just add 5% to 10% distance and intensity per week. You have the right to ease up on training every 4 weeks. This means returning to your training plan 2 weeks prior. After that, go back on track with your 10% increase per week. Again, after 4 weeks, ease up, then go back on track.

- Monday: Walk 3 minutes. Run 1 minute. Repeat 10 times
- Tuesday: Rest day or alternate training day
- Wednesday: Jog easy for 10 minutes. Walk 5 minutes. Repeat 10 times
- Thursday: Rest day or alternate training day
- Friday: Jog and walk depending on how well you feel. 50 minutes total.
- Saturday: Rest day or alternate training day
- Sunday: REST DAY (1 day a week is dedicated for zero exercise)
- Once every month, forego an interval run and change it to a WOD run (see chapter 11)

Chapter 6: Keeping Yourself Motivated

The first few months won't be a problem. You are still enthusiastic and/or stubborn about your weight loss program. After 3 to 6 months, you'll start to find excuses so as not to work out. The best way to minimize this occurrence is to:

Find a Running Buddy/Group

To be very specific: you want a running buddy who motivates you to work harder and hit the road. You don't want someone who is lazier than you! A running buddy/group also helps you push yourself more. This is because the pain on your legs is less noticeable when you are running in a group.

Reward Yourself

Set milestones, i.e. every 2 months. If you are able to run relatively uninterrupted by your laziness, for 2 months, then reward yourself with a sumptuous meal, or a dry fit shirt, or a nifty heart rate monitor.

Don't Push Daily

The 10% rule is there to stop you from going too fast too soon. It does not mean you should add 10% to your workout each week. If you want to take 2 weeks before you add 5% to your intensity and distance, that's okay too. The important thing is to steadily increase your distance and speed on regular basis.

Music Playlist

Strap on your smart phone and headset. Create a running playlist! Pick energetic songs that increase your rhythm.

Social Media

Most smart phones have an application that tracks your speed and distance travelled, and then allows you to post it on social media. Simply put, bragging rights can also be a motivation!

Chapter 7: Fast Metabolism To Burn Fat Fast

Granted, your metabolism is affected by your genes; but you can also tweak your metabolism with your lifestyle. Below are a few points to remember.

8 Hours of Continuous Sleep

8 hours of shut eye allows your body to repair itself. As a result you wake up refreshed and raring to go. This also means your body is not in "safe mode", resulting in a slower metabolism. There is also the fact that 8 hours of sleep make you more energetic. This means you are more preconditioned to exercise in the mornings or have plenty of energy left to exercise late in the afternoon.

Eat Breakfast

Skipping breakfast sends a signal to your brain. Your body tells your brain to go on calorie conservation mode the whole day. As a result your metabolism slows down. On the flip side, eating a healthy breakfast tells your body that there is food to consume. It then sends a signal to your brain that it can go for optimal performance, resulting in a faster metabolism.

Eat on Time

Eat your main meals on time. If you skip a meal, your body goes on conservation mode. If you are late in eating, your body is already at conservation mode. Hence you use less and store more fat.

Eat Smaller Meals

If possible, eat 5 smaller meals each day as opposed to 3 big meals. This has been known to boost your metabolism; and this minimizes the actual foods you eat because you feel full all the time.

Eat the Right Foodstuff

Yes, there are foods that are known as metabolism speed boosts. Think antioxidants. Then incorporate the following into your regular menu:

- Berries
- Almonds
- Cruciferous vegetables i.e. cauliflower, broccoli, Brussels sprouts, etc.
- Spicy foods i.e. chili
- Cinnamon
- Green Tea
- Whole grains
- Apples (especially in the mornings)

Chapter 8: Build Lean Muscle

Training your core allows you to run longer. It also allows you to run in proper form. By doing so, you burn more calories. When do you train your core and upper body? Look at the sample training plan above and refer to "alternate training day".

Proper Form Life Hack

It's hard to describe proper form in an eBook. The author can be correct and very specific, but the reader can't really understand everything. Here is a simple hack. Know the exercise you want to perform i.e. planks, modified planks, dumbbell curls, bicep curls, triceps curls, etc. Go to fitness gyms. Some even offer free 2 to 10 sessions! Now hire a trainer. Ask to be assisted with your target exercise. Listen very carefully! You can even ask to record the session for your blog.

And Wa-Lah! Now you have proper form and you aren't bothered by gym membership! Tip: try to return to the gym once every couple of months. Hire a trainer and check that you still have proper form.

Avoid Sit-ups

Sit-ups are among the most ineffective ways to train your core. It also has the tendency to result in back injuries. Avoid these altogether.

Planks

Planking is the way to go. You want to start with 30 second planks, rest 1 minute then 30 second planks again. Repeat the same 3 to 6 times. Your goal for the next few weeks is to increase your time 10 to 20 second per week until you are able to plank for 2 to 3 straight minutes.

Modified Planks

Modified planks should be done after simple planks. It should be done in succession without rest. Each position can be held for 10 to 20 seconds at a time for beginners. Typically, you start with a

30-second plank and then transition to arm raise left and right; leg raise left and right; side raise left and right; then finish with a raised plank for as long as you can.

Low Weight Curls

You want to start with a simple dumbbell or barbells without weights. Perform curls 16 to 24 repetitions for 2 to 4 sets. You start with 16 reps and slowly build it up to 24 reps within the span of 1 month. Now add some weights. After each month, you can increase the weights but never more than 10% each month. Remember, proper form is more important than repetitions or weight. So take things slow and make sure to avoid using momentum to lift the weights.

Swimming Frog Style

Swimming is a fantastic alternate core training regimen. Frog style in particular activates your hip flexors and pelvic muscles while at the same time building up your core and toning your arms. Start with 12 repetitions with 3-minute breaks after completing 1 lap. After each month, minus 30 seconds to your rest period until you are able to complete 24 repetitions without resting. Take this slowly, and complete the full motion of leg kicks and arm strokes.

Chapter 9: Recovery Days

The first cardinal rule is to always have at least 1 rest day per week. This allows your body to rest up and is also your reward for a job well done. This means no exercise whatsoever.

The second cardinal rule is not to work the same muscle group 2 days in a row. This means that if Mondays is running day for your legs, then Tuesday is core and upper body training day. By way of exception, you can warm up during your core training days with a brisk walk. This is known as a recovery walk or recovery jog. Make sure to take it very slow. If you have a heart rate monitor, you want your heart rate to stay within 55% to 60% of your maximum heart rate.

The third cardinal rule is to know the 2 different types of pain. The first type of pain is the regular type. Bear in mind that there is no such thing as zero pain running; but this type of pain can be characterized as mere discomfort. This usually goes away after 1 day of rest/recovery.

The second type of pain is the type that shoots thru your nerve and up. This also includes pain that does not go away after 3 days of recovery. When you feel this type of pain, you should immediately stop and take a few days off.

Recovery Swim

Going to the pool is good for your legs. This can be done 30 minutes after you jog and/or the day after. You don't need to do much. Just rest the legs; but you can exercise a different muscle group like your arms, hip flexors, pelvic muscles, etc. Simply being in the water helps. This is because the cold water soothes your muscles. The pressure of the water compresses your legs better than any compression gear; and your buoyancy lifts the weight from your legs without it being in a seated or lying down position.

Chapter 10: HIIT (High Intensity Interval Training) And WOD Running For Beginners

You can't help yourself, when you run you want to run fast. This is especially true if you are running with strangers and they're overtaking you left and right. You want to speed up! Let us help you with that!

3 Month Rule

Unless you're an experienced runner, you need to accumulate at least 3 months running 3 times a week before you attempt High Intensity Interval Training i.e. WOD running. By doing so, you prepare your body for the pounding it will take. Bear in mind that 3 months of running with proper nutrition is necessary to allow your body to:

- increase bone density, especially in your legs;
- increase muscle strength and durability; and
- increase your cardiovascular and lung capacity, resulting in faster recovery
- consistently run in proper form even when tired

What is WOD Running?

Simply put: you run at breakneck speeds: run, then rest, then run, then rest, then run. The catch is, for each succeeding run, you increase the distance and decrease your rest/recovery period.

The author suggests you start with a modified WOD. This means you don't go balls out. You run at high intensity, but lower than your fastest lap.

How Fast should you Go for WOD?

After 3 months of regular training, run 2 kilometers at a modest pace. Now run 1 kilometer as if behind you is an angry bull with sharp horns, trying to ram it in your bung hole. Make sure to time yourself when doing this. Your speed for the third kilometer is your WOD run speed a.k.a balls out speed. Minus 45 seconds from that speed and that is your modified WOD speed.

Modified WOD Training Plan

1. Jog 1 kilometer at moderate pace. (Don't forget to warm up before this lap!)
2. Run 500 meters to 1 kilometer at your modified WOD pace.
3. Rest for 3 minutes by walking slowly.
4. Run 700 meters to 1.2 km at your modified WOD pace.
5. Rest for 2 minutes by walking slowly.
6. Run 500 meters to 800 meters at your modified WOD pace

3 Important Requisites to Follow

   a. As you can see above, steps 2, 4 and 6 have two distances each. The first distance is your starting distance as a beginner. The second distance is the one you aim for, after 2 to 3 months of performing WOD. Again, remember the 10% rule.
   b. Time yourself starting from step 2, up to step 6. Minus your total rest minutes (5 minutes). The trick is to keep your running speed as even as possible. In other words, you aren't faster in step 2, slower in step 4, and slowest in step 6.
   c. When you are now able to perform steps 2, 4 and 6 at the maximum distance and at a relatively even pace, it's time to run at your balls out speed.

How Does that Help Me Race Other Runners?

Simple: if you are doing your modified WOD and WOD right, and keeping true to relatively even splits, then you'll probably be too sick of running fast. In other words, you don't really care who overtakes you anymore! When running, you just want to run at your own pace based on your training plan. Now you can really say, you're an experienced runner!

How Does WOD Slim you Down?

WOD, strains every bit of your body. If you do this in earnest, at the max distance, you'll probably be hitting 98% to 100% heart rate at the end of the last interval. As a result your mind tells your body to speed up its metabolism and eat up more fat and calories.

Tip: Again, remember to eat within 30 minutes after your run. However, for HIIT and WOD runs, it is better to increase the ratio of protein you eat by 10% to 20%. This is because at 98% to 100% heart rate, your body needs the added protein.

Conclusion

Thank you again for purchasing this book on The Ultimate Running Weight Loss Guide!

I am extremely excited to pass this information along to you, and I am so happy that you now have read and can hopefully implement these strategies going forward.

I hope this book was able to help you understand the correlation between a healthy running lifestyle and how to lose weight.

The next step is to get started using this information and to hopefully live your life to its fullest. Remember "SWEAT IS FAT CRYING!"-unknown

Please don't be someone who just reads this information and doesn't apply it, the strategies in this book will only benefit you if you use them!

If you know of anyone else that could benefit from the information presented here please inform them of this book.

Finally, if you enjoyed this book and feel it has added value to your life in any way, please take the time to share your thoughts and post a review on Amazon. It'd be greatly appreciated!

Thank you and good luck!

Preview Of:

Ultimate Mindful Eating Guide!

<u>Mindful Eating</u>

Stop Overeating And Binge Eating For Good And Lose Weight With Mindfulness, Self Discipline, Meditation, And Willpower Strategies!

Introduction

I want to thank you and congratulate you for purchasing the book, *"Mindful Eating: Ultimate Mindful Eating Guide! - Stop Overeating And Binge Eating For Good And Lose Weight With Mindfulness, Self Discipline, Meditation, And Willpower Strategies!"*

This Mindfulness Eating book contains proven steps and strategies on how to avoid overeating and binge eating for good. It is easy to fall into the trap of mindless eating especially given the world's culture today, but it does not mean that overeating should be a normal part of life.

Overeating and binge eating can lead to serious health problems and issues, and it is time that people take an active stance against such issues. Lead a healthy and well-balanced life by following simple steps and strategies that will keep you off your cravings and away from binge eating.

Thanks again for purchasing this book, I hope you enjoy it!

Chapter 1: What Does Mindful Eating Mean? What Does Binge Eating Mean?

Eating is a natural way of life. People, along with all the other animals and living things in the world need to eat or consume foods in order to grow and survive. However, there is more to eating than simply shoving up food into our mouths.

Mindful Eating

In the world today where food seems to be everywhere, the act of eating becomes what is known as a mindless deed. There is hardly any thought that goes along with the action and many people seem to just eat whatever food is right before them. In some cases, people are not even aware of the foods that they consume or would simply forget about them mere minutes after they have eaten. These facts tell us that the act of mindless eating is so rampant that it oftentimes leads to guilt and weight and health related problems. If there is such a thing as mindless eating, what is mindful eating then?

To some, mindful eating is the act of being fully aware of and in control of what they eat. This means that they pay every attention to the foods they eat and are therefore able to notice and enjoy every bite they take. It also means being aware of the foods' effects on the body, and therefore having the intention of taking care of oneself. After all, no one would mindfully eat something if there is a known negative effect on the self. To this respect, mindful eating builds a peaceful relationship with the body where the body's needs and sometimes even the wants, are satisfied. It becomes an act of wisdom and of full consciousness as it chooses what is natural and healthy.

Binge Eating

On the other end of the spectrum is what is known as binge eating. This is the earlier form of eating that was discussed as being mindless, and even sometimes taken to an extreme level. Binge eating is defined as disordered eating wherein the act is uncontrollable. This leads to eating enormous amounts of food even after the individual has had the feeling of a full stomach.

Most people who suffer from binge eating try to hide it from friends and family, leading them to isolate themselves in many instances.

In extreme cases, binge eating is a serious disorder where one consumes unusually excessive amounts of food. Even those who are not diagnosed with the disorder can experience occasional bouts of binge eating where they find themselves unable to restrain themselves from eating. In some books, the definition of binge eating is excessive and uncontrollable eating that is followed by feelings of guilt and shame. This compulsive eating disorder also leads to many weight and health problems including but not limited to obesity and excessive weight gain. Women have been found to make up 60% of those with binge eating symptoms and one in every five women have reported to experiencing symptoms of binge eating.

Thanks for Previewing My Exciting Book Entitled:

"Mindful Eating: Ultimate Mindful Eating Guide! Stop Overeating And Binge Eating For Good And Lose Weight With Mindfulness, Self Discipline, Meditation, And Willpower Strategies!"

To purchase this book, simply go to the Amazon Kindle store and simply search:

"MINDFUL EATING"

Then just scroll down until you see my book. You will know it is mine because you will see my name "Sarah Brooks" underneath the title.

Alternatively, you can visit my author page on Amazon to see this book and other work I have done. Thanks so much, and please don't forget your free bonuses

DON'T LEAVE YET! - CHECK OUT YOUR FREE BONUSES BELOW!

Free Bonus Offer: Get Free Access To The www.LiveFitVIP.com VIP Newsletter!

Once you enter your email address you will immediately get free access to this awesome newsletter!

But wait, right now if you join now for free you will also get free access to the "The 7 Keys To Body Transformation" free EBook!

To claim both your FREE VIP NEWSLETTER MEMBERSHIP and your FREE BONUS EBook on THE 7 KEYS TO BODY TRANSFORMATION!

Just Go To:

www.liveFitVIP.com